To: Meg

With best wishes.

Chris.

Nov 2011.

CHRISTOPHER J KNOTT-CRAIG MD

LEND ME A KISS

CHRISTOPHER J KNOTT-CRAIG MD

LEND ME A KISS

*A collection of short poems reflecting the Love, Pain
and Spirituality of a Pediatric Heart Surgeon*

Langdon Street Press
Minneapolis, MN

Langdon Street Press
212 3ʳᵈ Avenue North, Suite 290
Minneapolis, MN 55401
612.455.2293
www.langdonstreetpress.com

ISBN-13: 978-1-936782-36-9
LCCN: 2011935275

Distributed by Itasca Books

Cover Design and Typeset by Melanie Shellito

Printed in the United States of America

*This is for Dada's sweetie pie, Catherine Rae,
and for CIP (Connie the Ice Princess).*

CONTENTS

ACKNOWLEDGMENTS

No one encouraged me to formalize these poems more than my immediate family, especially my daughter Annie, and my brother Alan Knott-Craig.
And of course our insolent red Persian cat, Ginger. And no one enjoyed them more than my mother,
Andy Knott-Craig.

PREFACE

As a surgical colleague succinctly put it, pediatric cardiac surgery is one of very few professions where each day the surgeon goes to work with the real chance of his or her patient dying. Most surgeons insulate themselves from this emotional challenge with a cloak of professional indifference. For others, including myself, caring for these voiceless, defenseless, infant patients is more than a profession—it is a passion, which exacts a huge physical and emotional toll that is difficult to describe in words. Needless to say, the incidence of suicide, "accidental" deaths, and "burn out" of pediatric cardiac surgeons is amongst the highest of any profession. There have been many days that I, too, felt that the emotional toll was too high to bear alone.

These strong emotions—the passion and ecstasy of love or of a successful surgery, the depression and despair of losing a patient or of alienating a loved one—are nakedly portrayed in my poetry. I share my interpretation of the pain I see in my patient families: the pain of divorce, loneliness, obesity, or fighting addiction. The therapeutic friendship of family pets, the narcissism required to operate on another patient after losing a patient hours earlier, continuing to find new operations, new cures or palliations—these are evident for all to read. The anger at God for allowing my patient to die, the reluctant acknowledgement of His Divine wisdom, and the longing to grow nearer to Him are obvious.

Meri Armour, president and CEO of Le Bonheur Children's Hospital said it best: "You are high maintenance because you see everything in Technicolor — the blues are bluer, the reds redder, the greens greener. There is no gray in your mind." In many ways I stand naked before the literary audience, warts, scars and all. Why then do I want to share these poems? The answer is simple: not only does this represent a confession or purging of sorts, but reading them has been very therapeutic for me and many friends and family members who have felt these same emotions. Perhaps, you too will laugh and cry and find solace in the fact that you are not alone in your emotions. I hope so.

LEND ME A KISS

Lend me a kiss for the love I miss;
that I may know the pounding in my chest
is that of life, not the death
of my mind and soul.

Lend me a kiss and small embrace
and lay your breasts against my face
that I may feel once more the nurture
from which babes are fed and coaxed to sleep,
that I too may rest and feed my mortal self inside.

Lend me a kiss and keep not score.
Think not ahead of less or more,
not of remorse in days ahead;
but that in serving, pain is shed
and let gratitude suffice.

Lend me a kiss today.
Lend me a kiss, I pray.

BABY HEART SURGERY

It quivered just a little in my hand—this tiny heart,
and my soul soared!
With the quiver came a sliver of hope, of a chance
to live, or live again without pain
in this instance.

And as this limp pump came alive
part of me smiled but part of me died
of pride and shame,
of running the race and having to win
again and again and again.

WHILE YOU WERE GONE

It was cold and empty and quiet while you were gone;
there were no love calls from a dove,
no twittering of sparrows on the tree limbs above.
Even the wind waded through the trees
without rustling any leaves.
The tree frogs were mute at night
and the cicadas were silent
while you were gone.

I wandered around the house like a ghost.
Neither television nor movies could provoke life
to the shell I called home.
My heart was empty and my soul ached to be held.
And I thought it must be awful to die alone.
Neither wine nor down comforters
could warm my hands and feet
—or my heart,
while you were gone.

And I knew then
that home is not home
without you.

I TOUCHED YOUR FACE
WITH MY HAND

I touched your face with my hand
and traced the faint lines around your eyes.
Your skin was so soft under my fingertips.
I wondered how many tears had slipped
from your shuttered eyes and trickled down your cheeks
unseen, unnoticed, and undried.

I touched your face with my hand
and ached to hold you close
to kiss away that sadness—and the hurt—
caused by careless words—those present
and those from the past chapters of our lives.

I touched your face with my hand
as you touched my heart with your smile.
And I drew a line in the sand
and hoped the ocean's waves would not erase it
as it had before.

I FELL IN LOVE TODAY

I fell in love today with an unknown woman.
Later on I fell in love with a baby I operated on.
This afternoon I fell in love with a painting I never liked before.
Each time I breathed, love came out!
But from where?
You know what?
I don't care.

SONNET II

They're like a cherry on a summer's day
Or the wild speckled mushrooms in a field
Spreading conjured fantasy yet to yield
Or reach fruition with so much to say.
Spongy as untamed grass on rolling hills
Pregnant as a plump pod holding snow peas
Bursting to consume or devour with greed
Moistly mystic melon sans leather peels.
That these two halves can so completely heal
What from within has caused such pain to feel
But when invited opened wide they spread
Can melt the hearts of stone and mostly dead
That this be truth and truth as such be told
One kiss from you is all my heart can hold.

BABY HEART SURGEON

He smiled at me—
When he opened his eyes he smiled at me—
I cut his skin and broke his bones
and sewed and patched and closed the holes
in his tiny heart.

And then, when all was done,
I wiped away his tears with my thumb.
"You're okay," I hummed.
Then he opened his eyes and smiled.

This time it was I who cried.

GINGER

The red Persian stood there and stared at me.
His eyes blinked in slow motion as he flicked
his bushy tail from side to side in an irritated gesture
before he settled on his knees and purred outright.

"I am forced to wait for you to feed me."
"My coat is knotted and tugs at my skin
but you don't begin
to notice me anymore."
"Will you stay with me? Or go away
like everyone else I've known,
everyone I've loved inside this home?"

"Come here, Ginger," I purred,
and scratched his nose.
Scratched under his chin. And his toes.
He rolled on his back and bared his tummy
for me to scratch.
Content.
My Persian cat.

Happy to be loved even for just a moment
...just like me.

A FAVORITE COUCH

It's the surrogate mother
who beckons when you're so tired
it's an effort just to hold up your head,
or answer the phone, or pour a cup of tea.
When you legs ache even while you're sitting down,
it wraps itself around you like Nana's hug or an embrace.
It cradles you in that lazy fetal position.
allows you to let go, float away for a while
to Neverland
or some other place.

Everyone needs a favorite couch,
a go-to place to rest,
....or a friend.

DREAMS

Dreams are those friends
who are always there—
who understand that love and pain
are the coat and bowtie of the clothes we wear:
the red and white which fills the fluted glasses
in our hands, the day and night
inseparable yet opposite
as the clouds and air.

Dreams are friends
and friends may go their different ways
and dreams may fade into the night—
into the air, and still be there.

A HOLE IN THE SOCK

There was a hole in his sock
which no one saw or noticed.
It was not visible when he crossed his legs
or strode briskly here and there and everywhere.
It started as a tiny hole over his little toe.
Over years it grew, mostly unnoticed, except by a few
as it scratched and chafed
until one day in a rage
he took off his shoe
and threw it away.

Everyone was amazed
at the big hole in his sock.
Hidden and disguised for so long
like the words of a song
often hummed—but never sung
until now.

A LARGE BIRD SAT
IN MY GARDEN

A large bird sat under the tree—
just sat there and stared at me
and the pool and the garden;
I wished that there were more flowers for him to look at,
that I had cut the grass the day before,
and scooped the autumn leaves out of the pool.
But I was a busy person! I could not do everything at once—
some things needed to wait until I had more time!
Right?
Surely he could understand this!

Then I started to wonder...
what he was doing sitting under the tree
in my garden this Sunday afternoon
like a lazy farm laborer at noon,
or a poet with nothing to do or write about,
instead of sitting high up in the tree
like he should,
being an eagle and all.
I wondered if he was hurt.

Had he perhaps dropped his meal and was too embarrassed
to search for it with me watching?
Or was he just lonely and dejected like me?

I wanted to cry.
He wanted to fly.
Just him and me.

A SINGLE TEAR

A single tear rolled down his cheek
But no other tears rushed to join it.
His eyes never wavered in their faraway stare
and his lips were pressed in a straight line,
straight as a line in the sand.

"What is the cause of this tear?" someone asked.
"It is not a tear," he replied, "for tears imply pain, or remorse;
and I have neither.
Tears are the indulgences of the weak and the bored.
No, it is just a misplaced drop of salty water on my cheek,
nothing less, nothing more."

"But if it were a tear—which it is not—
it would come from the well of ache, not pain,
and dry into the air with the indifference
of a life lost in war.
Or a war within a war."
Or simply evaporate unnoticed
like before.

MY SAFE SPOT

It's soft and warm, smells like home.
I lay my head there and listen
to the vibrations of life resonating in my ear:
I could hear his heart beating when I was small
—even when I was less small—
Scratching my head, arms wrapped tightly around me
kissing my brow lightly as I drifted away.
Into my dreams.

Between his shoulder and his chest
below his chin and neck—
This was my safe spot
My happy spot
My home.

AT THE AIRPORT

Half dressed, all the carry-ons a mess!
No shoes, just awkward socks
surrounded by smelly feet
and starched bored uniforms
in this perpetual rush and heat.

Gloved hands roam the bags
feel and touch the bras and pants
which before were neatly packed.
And murmur "thanks"
All the while we fake a smile and look around.
We feel important waiting in our socks
for the chance to fly
First class (of course).

AT THE CLUB

Twirling in the candlelight,
rocking while the darkness triumphed
over the dimly lighted room and the weary waiters
and even more weary band.
The darkness could end the dancing.
And the dining could cloister the anger
and silence the whining,
but could not blanket the lights
over the city of Birmingham.

Neither could the darkness
dim the light I could almost see
but felt in my heart
with you in my arms that night.
That unforgettable night
at The Club.

NEW YORK CITY 9/11

Silence heard far away
mutes the cries of pain, and sirens;
teams of busy bodies strain
in their quest to stop the flow of death
in New York.
Numbed minds,
hypnotized
by the scenes before their eyes
empty, sickened.
What now? they ask
and stare at those
whose names are strange and hard to say.
As the dogs growl.

We search around
for someone to hug, someone to hold.
We bag our blood
yearn to share this ache
that tears inside our chest and sucks away our breath!
If only we could say, "Let's go"—and live again.

And then a song wells up from deep inside
and fills our heads and hearts
with those words which make us one:
"America, America. God shed His grace on thee!"

Finally we feel the choking tide of tears
at last set free—
we think of wasted life,
and numerous rooms and tombs
so prematurely laid
in New York.

THE BABY GIRAFFES

Those two child giraffes wanted to play with us
in the Bushveld on that early November day
on the plains of Africa.
They ambled over with their lopsided grins and oversized
ears, watched by their parents from the nearby thicket.

Yes, no doubt about it, they just wanted to play.
The Bushveld dawn mirrored the newness of their short lives.
They didn't even know us.
Yet they wanted to play—with us.

I wondered if they would still want to play
if they knew us better.

BEING OVERWEIGHT

Be absolutely still; do not move.
Not even a single muscle. Don't even breathe.
Now feel the peace this moment brings:
For an eternity you don't feel the rolls of fat
around your waist, the tightness of your jeans
or the pressure of your size-10 feet stuffed into
your size-8 high heels.

When you breathe again
the moment of bliss is gone;
you are again disgusted with yourself—
like yesterday, and the day before,
and like tomorrow.

BLISTERED HANDS

They were rough and blistered.
The skin was dried and cracked over the knuckles
of the long thin fingers empty of ornaments
or emblems of belonging.
The jar of cheap moisturizing cream
tucked away under the desk made little difference,
could not arrest the calloused pain in her hands
or erase the aching beauty in those azure eyes
and in my chest.

Yesterday she bushwhacked brush in rural Alabama
as if that explained it all.
Today she was an ICU nurse
helping patients with heart disease.

I held those hands in mine,
felt the tears hidden inside the blisters
of her life and soul.
I knew then
I had to make her mine.
Blistered hands and all.

BREAD PUDDING

We baked a bread pudding together on a Sunday afternoon.
It was during the winter months in Memphis.
We laughed and kissed
and stopped to dance in the kitchen
between adding the rum and raisins
and spreading apricot preserves over the French rolls
which we had neatly cut into one-inch slices.
Our love was hotter than the oven set at 400 degrees.
This was a time when nothing could stop our passion
bubbling over like champagne in a fluted glass.

It seems so long ago that we baked a bread pudding together.
So long ago since the passion evaporated
like the rum fragrance in the bread pudding,
like the Midnight Poison in your neck,
now that our sweetie pie arrived.

BREAKING UP

I smelled your scent in my bed,
held your empty wine glass to my cheek,
your prints still on it from the night before—
We had grilled mussels and salmon on the ground
and fired rockets of passion at each other this 4th of July
before we were wrenched apart by this unkind world
and the unkind persons in it.

I lit my candle one more time
and gazed at the pictures
framed with care before me on the table.
I sobbed as I looked at the loop you made
to hang my painting on the wall—
to remind me of your love
when you were no longer there.

I looked for you in each room, under every bed
before I realized you were gone. Out of my life
like the flame of the candle on the table
and in my heart.

CAN IT BE REAL?

Tell me how you feel
Which of this is real?
Will your smile light up a room tomorrow
as it lit up my heart today?
Will it stay, or slowly fade away
with the clouds that surround the sun?
then melt into drops of rain—
and cause umbrellas to open
in the faces and embraces
of lovers,
and others who feel the same?

Tell me how you feel.
Can this be real?
Such joy, such bliss
in a girl and boy
unless they are embraced
by Grace.

CLOSE YOUR EYES AWHILE

Close your eyes awhile and let them rest.
The roadmaps tell their story.
And your eyelids, heavy laden,
can't resist the flooding when you smile.

Close your eyes and let them rest.
Let them dry while shuttered from the sky;
drop the drawbridge to that spark and sparkle
which once did light a room and eye,
but now which covers closely like a womb
and bathes the little ones inside.

Once rested
they again will smile,
shine clearly, brightly,
with resolve and strength,
with a vision of a new world
—one with less pain.

COME FOR DINNER

Come for dinner.
We have the Good News
for an hors d'oeuvre,
Prayers for the main course,
And Grace for dessert.

We have a fantastic Waiter.
Let's have a feast—
I'm starving!

DAY DREAMING

Fly away little bird, little sparrow
from your precarious perch
on the narrow limb or tree of life.
Where are your chicks?
Where's your wife?

You sit and stare at the worms
at the seeds and the ants that surround you,
unaware of the danger all around you.
You don't see the owl
with his big eyes and his frown,
studying you with his sleepy eyes
from the safety of the treetop?
Pondering whether to catch you
or let you enjoy your view
for another day?

Wake up little sparrow
Wake up, I say.

DIVORCE

In a blink
the world changes
and I smell the stink—
the burned pages of my life.

In a blink,
tears cover my eyes
and I think
of all the goodbyes I need to say again.

In a blink
the view's erased;
that view which yesterday I craved
from which dreams and homes are made.

The book is closed.
So too the page
on which our blood was spilt.
So needlessly.

DREAMING OF YOU

I taste the longing in your soul
as I drank from the fountain of desire.
There was a quivering beauty to behold
and a smoldering furnace of fire.
I filled the space quietly
and felt the passion in your heart
with an abrupt eruption
which I had yearned for
from the start.

My chest moves slowly now
I feel your breath on my skin
and I begin to relax.
I hear your muffled sobs
as your guarded tears course down my chin
and dry saltily on my chest,
and wet
the string of beads around my neck.

It's late
and I wait for the dawn to arrive.
I'm alive.
Spent, but alive.

EVAN CHILTON'S HEART

➤─┤◆─○─◆┤─◄

I held it in my hands.
It seemed so tired, so limp,
so uninspired.
When I looked inside it was empty.
It had no more to give,
choked within the prison of her chest.

Within this sad bag of blood
I sensed a light still lit:
a pilot light of flickering faith,
of love and everlasting Grace,
and knew that God was there,
inside this dying baby's heart.

And so we cut
and sewed and built;
with His guidance forged ahead
in silence and in awe.
Then saw it stir, and come alive,
enthused and pump with zest
again.
This precious baby's heart.

We knew then there was hope and faith
in little Evan's heart. We also knew
that God was there.

PASSING GAS

I was sitting at my desk,
wondering what to do next
when the gas from last night's blackened redfish
startled me as it bubbled out through my pants.
I hoped no one in the office heard.
My anguish was replaced with a sense of pride
as I enjoyed the unique fragrance
I had produced inside.

I couldn't help but wonder whether my dog felt the same
when he licked his ass, then suddenly slunk out of the room
followed by my outraged nose—and shoe—
usually both too late to affect him or sanitize the air.
Then I realized there is something very satisfying
about passing a particularly smelly fart
for both man and beast.

And I wondered whether my dog would growl at me
if he were in my office right now.

(RACHMANINOV ROMANZA) DO NOT GRIEVE

In the empty night my heart wandered
like a stray cat looking for a piece
of discarded fish. Then my mind
caught up with my heart and said,
"It is time to go to bed,
to feed the dead
and almost dead."

My lips are dry, unlike my eyes;
my soul cries out silently
to no one in particular.
Music fills my ears but I cannot hear
except a stifled sob
from who knows where.

Then I look into my tea
I see a single tea leaf
clinging to the cup's edge,
and with a final gulp
I know it's time
to say goodbye.

DEAR GRANDPAPA

Dear Grandpapa, I miss you so!
You always seemed to know
what to say to make me feel
safe and happy in a way that I could trust.
I loved you—and you loved me, too.

I'm so confused
by my views
of who I am and what I feel,
of what I can and cannot do.
You listened and you smiled at me,
You told me stories of the goblins and the fairies.
Then I knew what was true.
Now I'm blinded
by all the distractions that surround me.
I miss you so, Grandpapa.

Come to me. Speak to me.
Hold me close.
Are you near?
Let me hear your voice again.
Can you feel my fear?

O, Grandpapa—I miss you so!

DEATH OF A PINE TREE

Death creeps quietly closer
finger by finger, toe by toe,
needle by needle
like the pathetic pine tree in my backyard.
Death creeps up not from without or from within
but here and there, pin by pin,
a mosaic of fallen branches—
ever-growing scars concealed
by a painted cosmetic appearance
covered, that is—
not healed.

Though the pine tree's bark remains intact
it's a comforting disguise—
a shroud to the gloom that looms within,
like wolves easily scared away
yet sneak back in smaller tighter circles
taunting their prey.
When the weariness sets in
the death bite's a relief—
painless by comparison,
scarcely real.

Where is that healing Son above?
or the nourishing Stream below?

Can the conifer not feel my fear?
Retired into oblivion
Not fight, not grow, not heal?
Being called to serve,
unwillingly it passed.
If only it could serve again.

"Take my hand and lead me on
through this life, and then beyond.
Cleanse me, wash me with your Blood.
Let me find myself in God"

Before I die for good.

A BROKEN TOY

A broken toy
he is just a boy.
His face will turn red
when you smile at him
or wink.

He can laugh. He can smile.
If you squeeze his tummy
his eyes light up and he says, "Yummy."
Now he has a broken nose
his tummy has been ripped open.

Will you then toss him away?
Send him to the farm
with the other broken toys?
Spent. Bent. Forgotten boys.
Or throw him in the fire?
I know…it's a quagmire.

FIGHTING ADDICTION

Another day
Another dream,
Will this be the one?
When the past is erased?
And the sun rises for the first time
on my resolve to stay dry in the rain?
This refrain which has echoed
so many times before.

But today is different
I'm determined to succeed
I'm stronger now.
I'm a lion.

I just need a little help
to get started today.
      —just a little one, I'd say.

FIREFLY

Firefly,
firefly in the dark,
you work so hard to make a spark.
When you glow did you know
for some—like me—that means "Hello?"

In the night
your little light makes me smile.
Do you know how you puzzle my cat
when you come and go like that
flying blind and then aglow?

You are like a star, just closer.
You let me dream
of love and other things
cloistered in my mind;
things safe which can't be found
or hurt by any star, or sound,
or light of any kind.

FIVE RED ROSES

I counted five roses in the vase.
Five red roses in a black vase.

The first rose crimson red
It stood taller than the others
—a tightly wound bud.

The second rose was less red,
its head drooped to the left.
It looked away from the rest.

The third rose
had a bouquet, a fragrant nose
and a creamy center— a double delight.

The fourth rose was widely open, also red,
its pollen clear for all to see,
waiting for a honeysuckle or a bee
to spread the seeds
and set them free.

The last rose faced right.
Smaller than the other four
not crimson dark, nor paler red,
seemed more fragile at the core
but for the thorns
which lined its stem.

I counted five roses in the vase.
Five red roses in a black vase.
On the mantelpiece
In the candlelight.
Of the Church
In which I sat
Alone.

FRIENDS DRINKING WINE

They sat around the table and laughed.

Laughed about the laziness of the farm laborers
sleeping in the shade of an oak tree.
Laughed about the sanctimonious prejudice of Baptists
hiding bourbon in their coffee flasks.
They laughed about mac 'n cheese
and how the limp noodles reminded them of their husbands
on a Friday night.
They laughed about Hilary stranded on an island
taking a bitch for a walk. Herself.

He had lost his job. She had lost her kids.
Another's husband was dying.
All this was happening in their lives
at the same time.
But they still had each other.
They were friends. The three of them
not counting the bottle of Merlot, that is.

And they laughed away the tears and the fears
that choked them at night
and deprived them of sleep
and the will to fight.
Within the group there was little pride.
But they would remain friends
even if someone cried
or went hungry,
or died.

FRIENDSHIP OF A CAT

He sat beside me on the loveseat
on the back porch.
It was late afternoon in early spring;
he had an itch under his chin.
So I scratched it for awhile
and his eyes closed in delight.
His tummy hurt from past fights
to stay alive—so I dug my fingers gently
in his side and rocked his bowels;
he groaned with pleasure
and hummed my favorite tune.

I told him I was scared of growing old
and he stared at me as though I was crazy.
I shared that I felt guilty each time
I ate dessert, or dark chocolate,
and he smiled. I hated the new rolls
of fat around my waist.
Ginger listened and looked briefly
deep into my eyes, then nestled closer
and stroked my hand with his cheek and whiskers.

We had a wonderful chat, he and I.
And I knew our friendship would last forever
whatever that means.
Or at least as long as we
both remained alive.

(Ginger died of cancer in 2009)

GROWING OLD

It's getting late, my Friend.
Come sit with me and let me spend
a moment to reflect, to recollect
your closeness, the magic of your spell.
I can tell when you're near;
You fill me with your strength
then set me free.
I am in You and You in me.

HAPPINESS

Happiness exists
where there is intimacy in thoughts and dreams
and the silence of shared togetherness,
where there is acceptance of the beauty
of imperfections seen and unseen
uncovered by the night or light,
blemishes nurtured in imagination
and in vocal and in silent wishes.

Happiness exists
when it's okay to differ—and both be right,
when you can equally enjoy the challenges of day
and the quietness of night, without anxiety,
when it's easy to choose the right words
to say you're sorry and what is right.

Happiness exists
when you are able
to be sad for a stranger's sorrow,
to feel the ache of an empty tummy
of a distant nation in a distant country,
to sense the anger and despair
of not knowing what and not caring where
help comes from:
a candy bar or a gun.

When coming third is winning gold,
when growing rich is growing old,
when keeping less and sharing more
is our nation's goal—not making war,
when each child has a mom and dad,
when warm is good and waste is bad—

That's when we will start to know love
and happiness.

HEARTACHE

How long does it ache
before a heart breaks?
How bad is the pain
before it's just all the same?
How cold is the night when the moon is dark
and the stars don't shine bright
anymore?

How lost is a loss
when you writhe and you toss
in despair, gasping for air?
And life seems spent
like a rose with no scent—and no thorns,
or a bull with no horns is a cow.
Meow, meow.

Yes, heartache hurts
like an unsatisfied thirst
like a curse.

HOW MANY KISSES DOES IT TAKE?

How many kisses does it take
to mend a broken heart
and make it right?

How many tears need to flow
in the quiet of the night when no one knows,
before my soul is purged of the fear
of being crushed again?
Before the moon and sun
both feel the same
with you in my arms?

How many hugs are there in an embrace
strong enough to keep away the cold
the frosty cold of indifference?
Strong enough to last forever to keep me safe?
To survive decay and age, and pain,
and all the same again
tomorrow?

How many times will I lie awake at night
and think of all the things I did wrong
before I can recall one thing I did right?

I AM A FLEA

I am a flea
On the collar
Of a Yorkshire terrier.

I am a fly
In an African hut
During summer,
Feeding on the dead meat
Hanging from the sky.

I am the high "C"
On a piano or a flute in Carnegie hall,
Created by the poor boy
Waiting for this chance
To create for an audience
A transforming marvel of joy.

I am the roof, the bricks and mortar.
I am everything I want to be
when I am with you.

I MET A FRIEND

I met a friend I hadn't seen for years;
we discussed how life changes
how one tends to forget.

We laughed at the times we had shared—
at how silly we could be:
like a flea on the back of a Persian cat,
making jokes only we laughed at
but didn't care.

But I was amazed at my friend,
at how much he had aged...
when I studied him carefully in the mirror.

I NEED SLEEP

Open wide and let me breathe into you
the love that consumes my body and my mind.
Let me fill you with myself, with the energy which flows
through my bones. That energy which now has dried up
and left me a limp fish in the market
waiting for the highest bidder to buy my body.

But, my soul is still free
and my spirit will soon dance again.
Dance the tango, or the salsa, or both, with you.
But first I must eat. And sleep.
And prepare myself for you.
Mostly sleep.

I SEE A BIRD FLY

I see a bird fly
Fly high in the sky
But do I dare wonder why?
Can I guess whether it is hungry? or scared?
Does it sing happily? Does it cry?
Then it disappears behind a roof
or a tree, or a cloud.
And I see it only for brief moments
as it flies up there in the sky.

How like that bird we are—
We too see only glimpses of each other as we fly
And our knowledge resides from these glimpses of the eye
as we rest to eat and sleep,
pauses from the times in our lives when we fly.
When we sing and fly
or cry and fly
or just fly.

I SEE YOU IN MY TEA

I see you in the rosebuds
red at the tips and yellow in the center
as they share their buttery scent
with those awake in the early morning,
when the dew glistens on their petals
like fresh tears of joy.

I see you in the night
with closed eyes deeply sleep;
I reach out and touch you next to me,
knowing that you are even closer
in my dreams than beside me
as you rest your head on my chest.

I see you as I suture an infant's heart
as I think of ways to outsmart
the brokenness of the organ at my fingertips;
and part of me wonders if you are smiling
as you peer over your computer screen,
a cup of Earl Grey tea in your hand.

I see you in the road ahead
as I drive home, my body tired but my mind wired for fun,
for a walk round the block—or a run.
The red car ahead of me

is your body swaying as you walk;
the truck beside me holds my hand
as we enjoy the sunset from the loveseat on the back porch.

I see you in my cup of tea
my soup, my salad,
the words I read and write,
the paint I brush on my life's canvas
and I long to be close to you forever.

I WONDER

And if I die will you cry?
I wonder.
Will the fountains of the earth
roar and flow with zest—or mirth?
And the wells of salty tears
harbors of such fun and fear,
will they, having served and wept,
now be dry, caked, and spent,
or nurtured by the bonds of love
cultured, coaxed by God above?
Sense not loneliness and despair
but the hope of fresh spring air—
recall the love amidst the toil,
smell the scent of fresh-tilled soil.

And when I die, will you cry?
I wonder.
Will you thank Him for the time we shared?
In a silent prayer will you tell Him that I cared?
so much for you, and Him.

IF I WERE A CAT

If I were a cat and you were a mouse
I'd chase you up and down the house.
I'd try to catch you but I wouldn't eat you
even if I were hungry.

If I were a hammer and you were a nail
I'd hit you on your head over and over again,
I but I wouldn't bend you in any way.

If I were a honeybee and you were a rose
I'd eat your sweet nectar with my beak and my nose.

But if I were a lion and you were an antelope
I'd lay down beside you and watch over you
as you drink from the watering hole we both know.
And you would be happy
And I would be safe.
at last.

I'M NOT ALONE—I HAVE A PHONE

I am not alone; I have a phone.
I can call my mom in the morning with my coffee,
call a friend with good news while at work.
At the gym I can choose whether to answer it
or pretend I didn't hear.
I can dial for a chance at romance,
call for take-out food to be delivered.

I'm not lonely. I'm not alone.
But I sure wish I could hug my phone.

IMPALA

He stood tall and arrogant and stared
unafraid yet well aware of the danger all around.
His tan coat was punctuated by black and white.
A crown of horns adorned his form.
Would they be thorns tomorrow?
He turned to show his back and the target
hunters could see as they took aim.

The impala, king of the Bushveld buck,
surrounded by the elements he loved
yet so alone in his anguish
here on his throne.

IN THE MIRROR

Who do I see before me?
I see me. I see a flea
that bites and spites and fights
for a chance to be free.

Who do I see before me?
I see a clown with a smile
painted over his frown,
who longs to be hugged,
and loved by God
even if he is just
a flea.

IN THE SILENT NIGHT

In the silent night my pounding heart
wakens my conscious senses; which, once aroused
torment the fragments of my mind;
which, if asleep, would allow rest
to creep up and stay awhile.

In the silent night there is a stirring in my chest,
a longing to be longed for,
an aching which food and moon can't put to rest!
Though the moon is full and bright
it grows smaller as the night stretches into day.
Not so the emptiness of my bed, and heart,
when you're away.
Away from me.

INSOMNIA

I cannot fall asleep,
cannot get comfortable.
I keep flipping channels in my head.
This sleepless rest is not enough.
It's a waste of time at best.
My mind flashes images of yesterday
and the dreams of tomorrow.
I wish I could turn off the switch.
Instead I relive anxiety and remorse.
I recall words too easily spoken
and gestures left unpracticed for too long.

As these pictures flash, I do the math
over and over in my head
instead of sleeping
as I should in bed.

KILIMANJARO

Fog descended like a blanket
shutting out the light and the footpath ahead
while we climbed on the saddle of Kilimanjaro.
We were overshadowed by doubt and rising panic
with our torch and fading batteries.
It was so surreal: a boat without a keel.

We were afraid to keep going,
more afraid to turn around,
suspicious of the sound of another voice
on the saddle of Kilimanjaro
and the wilderness of the mind.

Wanting to go home
Needing to be safe
Not knowing where
to find either.

KIRSTENBOSCH

Red-winged starlings soar and dive
down where the crimson Disa hides
in the crevice and cliffs
of Kistenbosch.
The rough blue Erica toilet brush
like adoring bridesmaids surround
the pink queen Protea.
The pincushions of the king
relish the view below
of the Cape flats, of Caulk Bay
and in the distance,
Seekoeivlei.

The haze and glare of the air
is seasoned by the ocean breeze,
scented by the snoek and mating seals
by the Hanepoot vineyards lust
and the Southeaster's sandy dust;
the view framed by shaded trees
stretches north to craggy peaks
and orchards of Ceres.

This is the hinterland of Rhodes
our beloved Cape of Hope
from the contoured slopes
of Kirstenbosch.

LIGHT ME A CANDLE

Light me a candle with a pale flame
to brighten my darkness and my heart
and warm both, though we're apart.

Pick me a petal of your favorite rose
which grows alone out in the cold,
where only the motherly moon
acknowledges the beauty of its red and cream bloom.

Taste me a chocolate soft and dark
that's come from the land of Stella Artois,
a truffle which will force my eyes closed
in bliss, like your kiss, when you're in my arms.
And I will show you a flame
which burns with passion in my heart
for you.

LIGHTNING STRUCK

It was dark outside and inside my head.
Heavy black storm clouds were everywhere in sight.
I could sense a torrential downpour coming
ready to overwhelm me and my cozy existence.

Then the lightning struck.
In the aftermath of the blindness which followed
the sun shone through surrounded by a halo
of gaggling geese and a skirt of colors, varying
from yellow to red to indigo.

Though it soon became dark again outside,
inside I could see clearly now,
and I knew where I was going.

LITTLE SPARROW

Fly little sparrow, fly
higher and higher in the sky
until you disappear from sight.
Your tiny beak pecks and cleans
darting here and dancing there
never resting, or so it seems.
Yet in the quiet of the night
when all things are asleep
you search within your nest for calm
and sing beneath your breath a song.
You smile and pray and help the sick
while your mate is working late.

So fly, my little sparrow, fly.
I will watch the sun and moon
until the morning when you return.

LONGING FOR YOU

>-I-♦>--O--<♦-I-<

I smelled your scent,
that unmistakable scent of love and loveliness,
of satisfied hunger of content.
I smelled it in my sleep
and knew you had returned,
that you had heard me weep
from far away.

I lifted my arms and reached out to you
without opening my eyes, knowing you were near,
sensing your surprise as I murmured your name.
I smelled your wet hair and felt your nose
touch my neck as you nestled closer.
My eyes remained tightly shut, afraid
that my sight would banish my lover into the night.
Like it had so many times before.
That is, before now.

LOVE

Love is young. Love is bold,
a steaming hot fire with smoldering coals.
The fuel of love is love itself:
The crooning of a pair of doves
The twinkling of the stars above
The smoldering embers burning low
in the sea-swept evening glow.
Stoic sparrows wetting their feet
waiting on sea-sand for a meal to eat.
Lovers walking hand in hand
on the firm part of the sand,
savoring the time, the touch,
the moment now at hand.

Precious as the night, and just as short.

LOVE IS PAIN

The measure of my love is pain, not joy
nor the frolicking of lambs in hillside meadows
nor the nuzzling of a stallion by a mare
with white-gloved hooves and chestnut hair.

Rather by the pain that rents my heart
and churns my gut until I hear your voice again
or see your smile
and taste the agony that separation brings,
that unrelenting fear of not being near you another day.

I'd rather die again, again
than live another day without you.

DON'T COMPLAIN

Don't complain about the heat
if you're a laborer in Arizona.

Don't complain about the flaky friends
you hang out with in a bar.

If you want fresh bread
go to a bakery.

If you want to be truly loved
meet my God.

MELANCHOLY

Staring in the darkness of another day
too sad to sing, too sick to pray.
Stumbling through the ruins
of my home and mind,
I'm blinking furiously
reaching out to anyone with a smile
or a compass
or a pile of nothings.

I Hear the music
I Feel the taste of red wine
on my palate, on my tongue.
But I can't see the label,
I can't find the table
or the chair.

Is there anyone there?
Anyone at all?

MISSED OPPORTUNITIES

Spring is in the air
and the adagio from Sleeping Beauty
Plays over and over in my head.
I open my mouth to sing but nothing happens—
no sound is made, just a croak
I'm thankful no one heard.

And I wondered how other many times
we miss saying something beautiful, something spontaneous,
perhaps even something silly—just because
we don't have the right words to speak
or the right notes to sing.
And so, we crawl back inside our cocoons
more afraid to try next time.

MUSIC OF THE SEA

Where is the sea, the surf, the spray—
the fresh sea breeze that starts each day?
The mist which veils the great expanse
of life, and love—of waves and sand?
The widowed sparrow's sandy prints,
the uncouth squawk of gulls on high—
orphaned snails with ice cream cones
burrowing to elude the tide?

Where is that fiery ball of light
that drifts beneath the waves at night?
That lights the moon and stings the stars
and comforts lover's trembling hearts?
Coaxing waves to spread out wide
with licking lapping salty tongues
clearing slates with each new tide
the past erased, new life begun?

The crashing surf and rocks that meet,
the song of sand beneath your feet:
fond music for the sea-sad ear—
it's there, it's here—listen, and hear.

MY CONSCIENCE

I need to feel free
to be good—or bad—
to be me.
I don't need a high. I don't have to be rude
Or nude. Or wild. Just free.
Free of these chains that strangle my mind,
and make it hard to find peace without remorse
Or guilt.
Just for a while
For this life.

MY PERSIAN CAT

My Persian cat looked at me with disdain
or so I thought at the time.
"Are you hungry?" I asked out loud.
"Do you want me to brush out your fur?"
"Do you need a treat? Is there a stink
in your parlor?

I picked him up and held him close,
snuggled my face into his coat of fur.
Then I heard him start to purr, louder and deeper.
Now he was content.
He didn't want "something" from me.
He just wanted to be held, to be loved.
Wanted a caressed kind word.
So I sat and held him a while
and ignored my cell phone
and ignored the time.

And I recalled how loudly you purr in those timeless moments
when we sit in silence and I stroke your fur.
And I wondered: if I tried real hard
could I still remember how to purr?

OBSERVATIONS
OF MY PERSIAN CAT

You're getting fat.
You come home late then drink some wine (usually too much).
You eat your supper way too fast and
you barely notice me before you go to bed—
I might as well be dead.
You don't look happy anymore, you rarely smile.
You no longer jog or golf with your friends,
don't seem to have the time.
If I could open my tin of food
without your help, I wouldn't care.
So I need to purr to show I'm there.

But I wish you'd sit with me a while
so I could show you the bird I stalked
and tricked and finally caught
behind a huge pile of leaves.
I wait for you all day.
One day you'll say,
"Where's my Ginger?"
And I'll be gone forever.

And you'll miss me
like I miss you today.

OUR FIRST QUARREL

The first time we quarreled I was sitting at my desk
talking to you on the phone.
You were on a bus returning from a conference.
The laughter around you made it hard to hear you.
I was mad at you: you were having fun, while
I was alone waiting for you to get back so I could tell you
how much I missed you when you were gone.

I called you names. And said many unkind things.
You said nothing back to me except that you loved me.
Later we met at the entrance to JC Penney in the mall.
You kissed me and melted away my anger.
And I bought a string of fake pearls from the store.
You were so proud of them
And I was so proud of you.

And I could not remember what I was angry about
anymore.

PALM TREES

The palm trees wave their malnourished arms
in the breeze, happy that they are not yet
part of another thatched umbrella or gazebo
shading the tourists' eyes from the sun.

When I pass by them, they beckon to me,
"Let me wave my freckled wilting limbs
one more day before they too are nailed
to a planted post in the ground
and left to die—like your Lord."

THE LION

I gazed at the lion as I sat and sipped
my tea on the Piazza Signorelli in Cortona.
He was guarding the Estruscan museum
sitting high up there on his perch, his throne.
He'd been there so long he'd turned to stone.
As long as I watched he never blinked
or moved or looked away,
this giant cat erect and proud
protecting things and beings long gone.

And I felt safe and secure with him there.
As I watched the crumbling contour of his mane
I ran my fingers through my hair. It felt the same.
Mostly faded
Mostly gone.

PRUNING TREES

You woke one day and started pruning the orchard,
the blossoms of the spring and the summer's fruits
that quenched your thirst and hunger, forgotten.
With sheers sharp as knives you went about your task
snipping, cutting, breaking until only its skeleton remained.
You had prepared the tree for another season.
You turned away and never glanced at the tree again,
never thought of the tree with its shortened branches,
its leaking sap slowly trickling down the trunk,
carrying with it memories of its former self
as it stood there weeping alone.

RECIPE FOR PASSION

2 ripe peaches
1 bowl of warm honey
2 hungry mouths
1 big unripe banana
2 probing tongues
4 soft busy hands
1 big bed

Bring above ingredients to a boil
then mix rapidly for 2 hours
let it simmer for 30 minutes
then mix slowly for another hour
and eat what is left over.

DOZING OFF ON THE BEACH

I counted 23 wooden stilts
on a pier on Ambergris Caye in Belize,
and four posts hoisting a thatch gazebo
at the end of this pier.
When I counted them again
there were only 22, so I
counted and recounted them
many times in the lazy afternoon sun.
Each time, before I got to the end of the pier,
my eyelids drooped and shut for a second
and then I had to start counting all over again.

I don't remember how many times I counted the struts
or how many there really were,
because when I counted them the last time
the sun had mysteriously disappeared and it was dark;
and it no longer seemed to matter
whether there were 23 or 25
or less.

SCRABBLE

Words just words
Herds of letters
Ferrets of feathers
Meaningless on a board
Scored but not accounted for.
I need more.
Show me the sack;
Let me feel your jack
Let me pack a queue
for you
tonight.

SEAWEED ON THE SAND

Dried sweat
dried grass
both arid and pungent
spat out by the sea.
The ocean's menstrual tide—
seaweed on the sand!

Beaded curly grass in a buoyant mass
pubic hair from the deep, a testament of past.
Steamy rhythmic clash, churned and lashed
Vomit of the waves
Seaweed on the shore.
Expelled by His hand
Later buried by the sand.

SEND ME A KISS

Send me a lark
that I might hear singing
good enough to drown the pain
of my own loneliness
and light a spark in my soul.

Send me a sunny beach
with sparrows tiptoeing in the surf,
prodding little bubbles in their search for worms,
with wispy sea oats coating the dunes
and pelicans snoozing in the bay,
where time and tide stand still—
unlike my life
which is slipping away.

Send me a smile. And a kiss
and a promise of more.
and a compass
to navigate this miserable abyss,
with which to find "North."

SHE IS YOU

She is the flame that lights my candle
on a dark and wintry day.

She is the salmon on the grill
on a perfect night at a perfect time
watched by the cat on the window sill.

She is the glint in the eye of a spider
when she spies a fly close beside her.

She is the fulfillment of a life
with abundant love, without strife.
She is me. She is us.
She is you.

SHE STOOD ACROSS THE ROOM

She stood across the room
pretty and secure, the allure
catching his eyes.
The pain of past mistakes
followed the sun to its sleeping place
and took with it her tears and sighs.

She stood beside him on the beach.
He took her heart and her hand
and filled the timer with new sand.
The fear of not being safe tomorrow
faded with the darkness as the sun
peeped over the drapes of the bed
she called her life:
A chocolate box of strife delights.

She stood with him silently and smiled.
He pointed to them both, the sun and moon,
the old man and the child.
Then he took a brush and held her hand
as she painted a new life canvas
for them both.

SHOW ME THAT YOU CARE

Don't say you love me
with a love which can't be real;
Don't tell me that you like the way
I often make you feel;
Don't whisper that I'm lovely
beautiful or neat—
Don't touch the calloused bruises
on the insides of my feet.

Tell me that you miss me when you're near and far away;
Tell me that you ache to hear my voice yet don't know what
to say;
Tell me that you love me

but show me that you care.

SOMEONE CAME KNOCKING

Someone came knocking at my door;
I covered my ears and closed my eyes,
to my surprise the knocking got louder:
Louder than my pounding headache
Louder than my racing heart
Louder even than that whisper
of indifference that choked me—
that I could see but couldn't change.

Finally, I answered the door
and You said, "Come to me!"

SOMETIMES I WANT
TO BE ALONE

Sometimes I want to be alone
like a rock picked up and thrown
left outside in a storm for the rain to wash clean
of the mud and grime
which clings to it over time.

Sometimes I want to feel the ache in my tummy,
that pain which I hide so well when it's inside,
hidden from anyone that is, except my pride.

Will someone ever stop to pick me up?
Dust off the sand and dirt
that makes me a quarry stone
no longer a river pebble?
Will someone wash away the hurt?

I want to be taken home;
I really don't want to be alone.

SONNET I

Her laughter gurgles as a brook
bouncing off the tombstones of my soul.
Her eyes huge almonds sad yet bold
beacons of compassion, nought mistook.
Crimson ripened rosebuds moist with dew
stretch lazily to a smile a chasm wide
inviting trembling trusting guests inside
yet guard the pearls within of ivory hue.
Within this Rodin-sculptured countenance
an untamed spirit and fountain of all love resides
mystic as that rainbow to behold not hold with hands
and gently nurtured as the stamen in the rose abides
so healed are hearts and angels in distant lands
and dreams are dreamed once more before they die.

SONNET III

Kiss not this face as friends do when they meet
Or brush this brow with such indiff'rent care
That in my sleepless sleep I sense you're there
Nor can recall it was my brow or cheek.
Let not your lips so gently touch my face
And eyes averted, turned away, resigned
Expect no smile or careless kiss in kind
That there be no receipt of this embrace.
But place a lingering kiss upon these lips
And quench the thirst within with gulps not sips.
Let taste and smell be allies to the skin
As trembling lips meet trembling limbs within
So that the passion which does course these veins
Within our lips and breath may burn the same.

SUNRISE

You could sense it before it arrived.
Almost smell it. Certainly feel it.
The forbearer of something good
something bright,
like the smell of freshly baked bread
as you enter a home with a bake in the oven.
Faint yellow half-circles turn crimson red
Humpty Dumpty from my vantage point in bed.
In silence he arrives and shoos away the demons
a psychedelic phenom
of glorious light.

TAKING A STAND

I am shouting in a storm.
My brain tells me no one hears me
and looks at my choices and fears
as I gaze from my balcony
and dream of flying away to a gentler world.
But I need to say goodbye
to those who don't seem to care,
who cannot hear the cries of my soul
or the sobbing in my heart—the part
that can't go on and can't return
to my safe place, which is gone.
From now on
I am a whore to life no more.

TELL ME WHY

For me to live, you must die. But why?
Can the worms and the ants
not feed themselves, not enhance
their lives without me?
Can a spider slip inside her
without the prize of a fly?
Someone tell me why!

Why does sweet wine turn to sour?
Why do we need to pick a flower?
Why does the frolicking young bull
have to die to make us full?
Or the joy and pain of birth
end in senseless death and curse?
Why does the rainbow disappear
when at last you're getting near?
For God's sake tell me why?

Why do I feel this pain
when I walk these streets again?
Why do I want to cry?
Is it because it is I
who needs to die?

THANK YOU

Thank you for the years we shared
for the moments I felt sure you cared,
when the pain left my chest
and I could soar in the wind
without effort.

Thank you for letting me love you
as I longed to be loved,
a teacup filled with chai
a touch of your hand
and a smile which promised more,
or a cheerful hug or "hi."

Thank you for the moments
when I could forget who I was not
and live in peace
with who I am.

THAT ELUSIVE BEAUTY

I watch you standing
in front of the mirror,
turning your face this way and that
as you paint your mouth and eyes
and apply more powders and creams—
Trying to sculp the beauty I see so clearly
when you lie asleep, your head against my chest
naked of all bottled glows
and all pretenses.

THAT QUIET PLACE

It's late and the sun is slipping fast
beneath the Alabama plains,
dragging with it my emotive soul
to that desert where even the wind is still—
before the cicadas start their frantic panting,
before the tree frogs croak their love songs
to anyone and everyone who would listen,
to that halfway place
where those alive realize they are dying
and the dead rest before going to bed,
that quiet place
where I can hear my heart cry
with the ache that severance brings
after so many years.

THE BATH TOWEL

You are still damp and your comb is ruffled from earlier.
You look so happy—spent but satisfied and happy—
like the lover whose naked skin you caressed
drinking her pleasure, drying her treasure,
stroking her hair.
I smell the Midnight Poison on your coat
and I can hear your smartass mouth and laughter
when I cover my face with your fabric
as I dry my tears.

I am jealous of you:
she lingers with you in her arms
yet leaves me all too soon;
stays on you, in you
as I ache to linger inside you
when you're here with me.

THE BOX OF FLOWERS

I received a box of flowers today
from a most unlikely person.
It had a simple yet touching note attached
which said I would be missed—very much.
I stared at it at length before unwrapping it
and reflected on my rushed existence
and unfulfilled intentions.

I thought how happy I could have made
many people if I had told them
that they would be missed, too.

THE BLUE CADILLAC

I gazed out the window from my fifth floor office
watching the cars traveling up and down 6th Avenue.
Some were speeding and swerving through the traffic.
Some were hesitant, unsure where to go.
A blue Cadillac stood on the side of the road—
It was beautifully washed and polished;
the wheel trims sparkled in the sunlight.
I expected it to race off down the road
but it was out of gas,
could not go on,
waiting for someone to fill it.

I often wondered
what it would feel like to be a Cadillac—
Today I knew.

THE DOVE

It was a dove
cooing gently
intently
as it flew above
the ruins of my life.

It spread its wings
dropped packages of things
to mark its territory
indelibly
in my heart.

I reached to touch it
wanted to fly away with the dove;
but part of me was afraid
this was an escape and not love.
It cooed softly. Cooed urgently
My little dove.

THE ELAND

He just stood there. Didn't run.
Didn't ruffle his back nervously.
He just stood and stared at me.
Curiously amused—
like a woman who'd been used
or abused again.
His eyes as gray as his sleek coat
hanging like a shawl beneath his throat,
the Eland—the biggest
of the antelope.

He dared me to shoot him
as he looked me up and down:
at my creased pants and sweaty teeshirt
covered in Bushveld dirt and grime.
You bet I shot him. Not once but twice
for exposing me and my cowardice.
I shot him good.

Then drove away.
my camera still in my hands.

THE EMPTY HOLE

There is a little hole
that I cannot seem to fill:
Godiva chocolate doesn't help.
Ravenswood zinfandel doesn't help.
Working long hours makes it worse
—once the tiredness wears off.
Running hills for an hour or two
or writing down how I feel
just makes me more restless
more aware of this empty hole
in my tummy—in my chest.
It's a relentless itch I cannot reach.

Yet I wonder,
Am I afraid
to scratch in the right place?

THE FACE OF NAVARRE BEACH

I smiled at the old man.
His face was powdery white;
there were tufts of silvery hair
here and there
on his balding crown,
a frown separating lines of stubble
from his cheeks and chin.

I smiled at the old man as I walked over his face,
tracing the furrows of his countenance
with my big toe
in the sand.

THE GARDENER

He cut the trees and spread the dirt
around the shrubs and flowerbeds
of his lot. But he forgot
to plant the seeds—
those seeds from which blossoms grow
whose fragrance and whose luster
is a show
in spring when we all know
sparrows are tempted to sing
and April showers mostly bring
rain and pain,
and more of the same,
unless the Son cultivates new seeds
and orders them to bloom.

THE GIFT

Tingling with anticipation he takes it out—
She gasps, and strokes it lightly,
its smooth shiny length distinctive, regal.
She takes it in her hand stroking gently
up and down and sighs excitedly.
Its head is ready, so full of promise
A drop spills from the tip
and courses down its length
onto the softened cloth in her hand—
the color unique, so different from the rest.

Thank you, my love, she murmurs,
for my Mont Blanc fountain pen.

ABORTION

I told an old man,
a stranger with kind eyes and soft hands,
about my pain—about the life I lost
and the price, yes, about the cost.
That empty hole which had been filled
with a part of you—with a soul I loved
and love even more today.

I told him how I prayed then, and pray today
that you would recognize my sacrifice,
how much I cared for you.

I told this to an old man—I told my father
and my Grandpapa
I told my God.
He never listened then.
Perhaps you'll listen now.

THE MISTRESS

I breathe his breath
and taste his kisses in my heart.
And part of me shudders with delight
and part groans with fright
for the caresses my body misses
but despises in the night—
when I awake and find he's not there,
and think he doesn't care—
to share the hell I live in
tossing and turning in despair.

Yet I hear him whisper in my ear
that he is here. And will be here for me...
I feel his fingers gently teasing now
that secret space between my thighs and brow;
His lips and tongue now urgently explore
the wetness of my soul, and I implore
"I am a fallen woman, just a whore!"
Yet in my heart I feel this heat
I haven't felt before. And lest he stop, I beg again
to bring me that mountain I adore
and let me see the heaven and the hell
from which once before I fell
and swore this mortal pain no more.

On my breasts the sweat has dried.
So too has caked the tears about my eyes.
And I am free of him. And yet,
I can't forget the sadness in his smile.
And I know...
it was worthwhile.

THE MOON AND I

You are an imposter, my friend.
I have watched you closely for many years.
I see you as you really are—all pretend.
I watched you as you grow and wane,
sometimes dark and just a smile
at other times a whitewashed ring.
I longed for your energy as you reach out to the stars
drawing them closer to you
like puppets on a string.

But you are just a reflection of the sun
Not real—just a dream,
—a face reflected in a stream.
You can grow bigger, but cannot come alive
without the Son. You and I both.
We are both lifeless.
The moon and I are one.

THE MOON CLOTH

She gave him a linen cloth to keep at his side.
It had red streaks on it, menstrual excess
like the streaks of tears which ran down her cheeks
when they said goodbye.
It came from a time when the tide was high
and the turmoil inside mirrored the bliss in their lives.
It would serve as a reminder
of the painting of their lives.

She gave him her moon cloth
keep him safe, to keep him dry
until he returned to her.

THE MORNING AFTER

The oak tree looked the same:
Tall and strong, arms stretched out wide
wrapped up in leaves and shade.
It seemed the same as yesterday.
It was not—
nourished with rain and dew,
warmed by the rays of a loving sun.
It had grown, imperceptibly matured,
was more alive than yesterday.
Though it looked the same
to almost everyone.
Just like me the morning after
I gave my heart to God.

THE NOSE

A nose is gross.
But do you suppose it knows
that it gets in the way when we kiss
or hiss or even sniff?

That it blocks our eyes
when we peep or spy on another?
That the smells it notes repels or quells
our thirst for love—
like the droppings of a dove?
Yet, when it's wet with tears of despair
that you're away and not here,
then it shows that you care
all the same.

THE OLD GUITAR

There is an old guitar in the study,
leaning back in its stand
waiting to be stroked, waiting to be played.

The room is indifferent to its potential
to light a room and raise the mood of those inside;
its mystic beauty and lacquered coat go unnoticed
like a painting on a bell or an angel locked in hell.

An unused guitar in an empty room.
A bride without a groom.
A dream without a soul.
Un-alive. Unappreciated. Fallow.
That is—until now.

THE PAIN OF LONELINESS

I look around and see such loneliness and pain
and relive what I felt so many times before—
an empty hopeless void,
a room without a door.

My soul aches as I fill another's void,
show I really care;
no one notices that inside
it is I who is in despair.

My heart cries out but no one hears.
Outside the clouds have hid the moon
I can't see where to go or who to fool
with my smile and confident demeanor.

Inside I long to be held
for who I am,
like a favorite toy
or a man.

THE PINE TREE

There were many pine trees in my front yard,
tall and straight, tightly crowded together
each stretching to outreach the others
to be the first to feel the sun's rays
and taste the breeze before it was dispersed
by the foliage of the others.

One of them was dying.
The needles on its limbs were brown
and less vigorous than its neighbors.
It seemed bled out, empty of all nourishment.
I hadn't noticed it before,
until it was too late.

I was sad for the pine tree
I was sad for me
I too felt bled out—
and wondered if anyone had noticed.

THE REWARD

He glanced at her tenderly
Full of expectation, overflowing with desire.
But she was not yet ready to engage.
He waited patiently and sighed—
This was going to be good
He had waited too long for it.
She was hot, so hot.
He anticipated her passion—
She smelled delightful—a mixture of
cinnamon and cardamom and ginger and mystic musk.
Finally she breathed, "I am yours, all yours."
He breathed deeply and reached for her.
He lifted her to his lips and tasted the richness
of her body, of her inside,
as he drank a cup of chai tea
from his favorite mug after a hard day.
Fantastic.

THE SEAGULL

On one leg he stands
in a trance.
Seeing without looking
at the sea, at the surf
for a chance
to feed
or maybe for romance?

He stands quite still
like a quill in the hand of an empty writer,
or an empty gun in the hand of a fighter.
Fly away, little fella;
you're not fooled by the sea
or the worm
or the weather.

THE TANGO

The long sleek forms melt and join
four feet above the sanded wooden planks
of the smoke-filled sultry club.
Through the cigar smoke and blurred twilight
and guttural sensuality of the moment
the notes of an accordion and a solo violin
seem to fuel the languor of the pianist
whose eyes are closed, as he sways to the rhythm only he
can feel,
except for the dark forms gliding around the room
cheek to cheek, chest to pointed breast
dispassionate and erect, like brooms.
Legs stalking each other with measured steps
stroking the black-clad man's inner thigh
with a polished shoe or a fishnet stilettoed ankle.
Exuding and the unmistakable promise of more—
much more, when the tango ends.

THE TORNADO

The dark clouds hung like sheets from the sky.
The whining of the sirens grew louder and louder.
Voices over the radio warned people like myself
to get out of harm's way. To hide.
The gusty winds had now subsided. There was
a sinister pseudo-quietness prevailing
and a sense of inevitability and of doom.

Although the tornado never touched down
The destruction that followed it
was evident everywhere!
That is, everywhere I looked:
Inside my heart.
Inside my soul.
And the ache I knew before
started all over again.

THE WINDOW

Shadows frame the window to the sky;
I am afraid to look outside
lest I die,
or wish to fly away.
I'd like to sneak
a little peek
through these shutters of the eye,
to see what's inside these pigeon holes.
But I wonder—
could I find my way back
once inside?

THE WORLD IS FLAT

From the window seat of the plane
the earth below is flat like a hat
squashed at the bottom of a suitcase
or a punctured bicycle tire,
a beer left open for too long
—quite flat.
The mountains and valleys look the same.
They are no longer high and low,
just a patchy-colored carpet below;
the lake's a watermark from an overturned glass
or an old cat waiting to die, leaving his urine stain
to mark his part of history
before he comes to pass.

The world is a squashed hat
a faded tattered mat
trodden on for too long
by too many wrongs.

Or so it seems to me.

THOSE SPECIAL WORDS

She said them softly in his ear
so no one else could hear.
He wondered if he heard it right
if he might have wished it said.
Then she said it again
whispered more softly this time.
But he heard it more loudly than a band playing jazz
louder than the ocean waves
crashing on the sand:
Those words—"I love you"

And he knew he would never be
as happy again as that moment
or more alive,
even if he survived.

TIME TO DECIDE

It's too late
for a date
to see if you care,
or feel safe with me.
To share.
It's too early to know if the hummingbird
loves being close or is just enamored
with the snack on the post.

But it's time to find out
if it's spring or fall,
if there's a roadmap ahead
—or a wall.

TODAY I AM TIRED

Today I am a limp fish
lying on a table at the market;
I have nothing more to give.
It is hard even to breathe.
I lie there panting while people prod me.
With great effort I squeeze my bowels
onto their hands, and, satisfied
wait for the journey home.

TWO EMPTY CHAIRS

Two chairs, yellow and green
side by side, one of each
at the high water mark
on Navarre beach.
Empty in the early morning

Were they occupied last night?
In the moonlight
when the tide was high
high like the passion of the terns
dropping recklessly into the sea
from the sky?

Sandpipers and plovers line up beside the chairs.
Some hang out in groups staring at the emerald surf
pensively contemplating life with one leg tucked up
under a skirt of feathers,
mouth hanging open in amazement
at the silver fish jumping out of the ocean
ready to be a meal.

White crabs peep out of their sandy burrows
puzzled at the plastic towers in their backyard.
Crabs and worms and mollusks of all sizes
on this perfect calm day on the beach.

The gentle lapping of the ocean
cleaning the sand for us to walk on.
Tea in hand, barely awake
erasing yesterday's numerous mistakes.

Two empty chairs.
Salt without pepper.
Love without a lover.
Us without each other.

WAITING UP FOR TEENAGERS

The clock has stopped I'm sure!
Look. Do you see the big hand's arthritic
and the little hand's stuck on three
like the simmering pot that won't boil the water
for my umpteenth cup of tea?

I imagine the headlights swaying and drifting
in the cursed half light of this endless night.
My heart is numbed with fright
waiting, starving for the phone to ring
or the sun to light the skies and lift
the weary eyelids of my teenager
driving home in his car.

WATER ON A TIN ROOF

Water keeps dripping on the tin roof.
Each splat is amplified beyond endurance,
bouncing off the insides of my head,
tap-tapping on the basement of my eyes
filling up my insides
with bile.

An unrelenting tide of scorn
opens that dungeon seldom visited
whose musky secrets stay locked
and hidden from all
both conscious and asleep
buried deep for so long.

That ache to fly again
and purge the pain of sin
surrendered now and limping
no longer proud or bold
but distant and aloof
and hollow
as the drip drip dripping
on that tin roof.

WHAT HAPPENED?

Where is the sun whose warmth embraced me
only yesterday?
Where is the sky that filled my life with so much wonder
that I never stopped to ask "Why?"
Where is Ginger, who listened to my whines
was my friend sitting on my lap,
who loved the sunset as much as I?

Just like the oysters we ate last night,
and the salmon we nibbled on as we laughed and loved;
just like the pinot noir which filled our palate with erotic
pleasures,
it all turned to piss and shit—
just like our lives.

WHEN THE BLEEDING STOPS

What happens
when the bleeding stops?
when you're all bled out?
How can a wound heal
without life, or nurture
without a meal?
Without a nurse, without blood
without a caring touch
without love?

What happens
when the bleeding stops?
If the heart still beats
and the Lamb still bleats
in the pasture, in the streets.
If there's a growl from an owl
or a miniature Yorkie
There's still life.

But how do you find it
without God?

WHO AM I?

Who am I? I seemed to sigh
when sea and sky are one;
and blue is sad and not the shade
I see here in the sun?

The gentle waves do comfort us
and with the spray they share:
the fleeting fate of life, of man—
from rain, to sea, to air.

Within this timeless beauty beach
created by His Hand—
I am a drop of salty sea,
I am a grain of sand.

WHO BLEW OUT THE CANDLE?

Two hands cupped around the candle
the tiny flame was so vulnerable
flickering and bending as the breeze nudged it
to the brink of extinction.
As the hands encircled it protectively
the heat from the flame scorched their skin
but the flame grew stronger.

Then an unexpected wind
from an unexpected direction
penetrated the protection
snuffed out the flame.
What a shame!
What unnecessary pain!

Who will light this candle again?

WHY DOES THIS EYE WEEP?

Why does this eye weep
on this cold and frosty day?
Dare I say
because it searches for, yet cannot find,
the sheep or hear their bleat
or that of the Shepherd's call.

Is this that tear of aching pain
which yesterday was shed in laughter?
Was the same
that lifted spirits high
that soared and roared
with eagles in the sky
uncatchable in its embrace of fate?

Or does it bleed from wounds not new or old
but from the wind and cold
of indifference?

WHERE BEAUTY DWELLS

Not in the heart clothed
with passion and with pain.
Not in the face which shines
and glows in life, or shame.
Not in the breasts warm and tender
though they be,
tingling in anticipation
of the wind and sea.

It's in the soul
and the sweetness of each breath we take
that beauty dwells
and dwells for all to see.

ABOUT THE AUTHOR

>→◆>-O-<◆><

Christopher Knott-Craig was born in rural South Africa in 1953. By age seventeen, he regularly helped his father as a sports correspondent for national Sunday newspapers *Cape Argus* and *Die Beeld*. In 1973, his first poem was published in the *University of Cape Town Christian Pamphlet*. He became a physician in 1977, and in 1986 was board certified with a Master's degree (summa cum laude) in cardiothoracic surgery, launching an internationally recognized career in pediatric cardiac surgery.

In 2004 *Christian News Journal* published his essay on "Miracles in Medicine." Compassionate pro bono cardiac care for underprivileged children in Africa earned him private audiences with Pope John Paul II and President Nelson Mandela.

In 1994, Knott-Craig made international news by performing the first successful repair of Ebstein's anomaly in a newborn baby, a hitherto fatal congenital heart condition. This procedure was done in Children's Hospital of Oklahoma while Knott-Craig was professor of Surgery at Oklahoma University.

A self-proclaimed rebel of the status quo, Knott-Craig introduced, in 2008, "Every day should be Valentine's Day," a novel family-orientated approach to pain-free cardiac care for babies with heart disease at Le Bonheur Children's Hospital in Memphis, Tennessee, where he is chief of Cardiac Surgery, co-director of The Heart Institute, and professor of surgery at the University of Tennessee.

His personal life ethic "The body is servant to the mind" is evidenced by his running sixteen marathons, climbing Mount Kilimanjaro (29,340 feet), and conquering his fear of heights with sky-diving. Other activities of interest include writing essays and poetry (in both English and Afrikaans), painting, and giving inspirational lectures.

Knott-Craig lives in Memphis with longtime friend, Connie, and their daughter, Cate. Their Persian cats, Caesar, Oliver, and Ginger, have all passed as a result of cancer.

He welcomes your feedback:

Christopher J Knott-Craig
741 Valleybrook
Memphis, TN 38120
ckc1132@gmail.com